THE GLYCEMIC INDEX & GLYCEMIC LOAD COUNTERS FOR 550+ FOODS - WITH A LIST OF THE TOP 330 LOW-GI FOODS

DR. H. MAHER

❄ Created with Vellum

INTRODUCTION

THE LOW-GLYCEMIC DIET IS A POWERFUL DIET WITH PROVEN results in weight loss, weight management, diabetes control, diabetes prevention and heart disease. It provides an eating plan and general dietary guidelines based on how foods affect your blood sugar level.

The glycemic index (GI) was originally developed in the early 1980s as a method to scientifically determine how different foods containing carbohydrates — vegetables, legumes, fruits, processed foods, and dairy products — affect blood sugar levels. Since that initial research led by Dr. Jenkins took place more than 35 years ago, many scientists have come to identify the opportunity that the glycemic index (GI) can be a powerful tool for maintaining weight, improving the effectiveness of weight loss diets, and managing diabetes.

The glycemic index isn't formally a diet in the sense that you have to conform to strict rules, follow particular meal plans or eliminate some foods from your daily meals. Rather, it's a scientific method of identifying how carbohydrates in foods affect blood sugar, levels, and measuring how slowly or quickly the carbohydrates in foods raise blood sugar. Thus, the

Glycemic Index referential is particularly important to know if you want to maintain weight, lose weight or if you want to take more control on diabetes, and certain health issues.

The "glycemic index (GI) diet" refers to a targeted diet plan that uses the glycemic index as the primary and only guide for meal planning. Unlike other dietary plans that provide strict recommendation with specific ratio, the glycemic index diet (GI diet) doesn't specify the optimal daily number of calories, the amount of carbohydrates, protein or fats for weight maintenance or weight loss but provides an effective eating plan with more flexibility and sustainable results in term of weight loss, weight management and diabetes control.

WHAT IS THE GLYCEMIC INDEX?

The glycemic index was first created in the early 1980s by Dr. Jenkins as a way to help people with diabetes gain effective control and management of their blood sugar. The original work consists of analyzing 60 foods and measuring how slowly or how quickly foods induce rises in blood glucose levels. The glycemic index is essential for health because a high increase in blood glucose levels can cause kidney failure or cardiovascular disease. Foods that have low glycemic index are known for their property to release glucose in the blood slowly and regularly. Conversely, Foods that have a high glycemic index are known for their property to release glucose rapidly.

Since that initial work, researches found that foods with a low glycemic index (LGI foods) are ideal for weight loss diets and foster weight loss, in addition to their positive effect on the pancreas (insulin release), eyes, and kidney.

The glycemic index (GI) is formed by scale from 1 to 100. Each food gets a score on this scale according to experimental data. A lower score indicates that food takes longer time to raise the blood sugar levels.

Complex carbs are superior to starchy carbs and refined carbs in term of weight loss and weight gain prevention diets. A pertinent differentiating criterion to choose healthy carbohydrates in based on their glycemic index.

Understanding GI values

Glycemic index (GI) values are divided into three categories:

- Low GI: This category comprises foods that have their GI value below 55
- Medium GI: This category comprises foods that have their GI value in the range 56 to 69
- High GI: In general, this category must be avoided because foods cause high spikes in the blood sugar level. Their GI value are equal or higher to 70

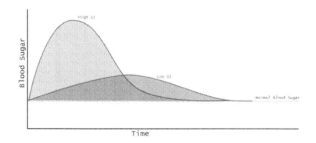

Comparing the GI values may help guide your food choices. For example, a muesli has a GI value of 86 ± 4. A Smoothie drink, banana has a GI value of 30 ± 4.

How Is Glycemic Index Measured?

Glycemic Index values of foods are measured using valid and proven scientific methods, and cannot be guessed just by looking at the composition of a specific food or the nutrition facts on food packaging.

Thus, the GI calculation Follows the international standard method, and provides values that are commonly accepted. The Glycemic Index value of food is calculated by feeding over than ten healthy people a portion of the food object of the study and containing fifty grams of digestible carbohydrate and then measuring the effect for each participant on his blood glucose levels (blood glucose response) over the next two hours.

The second part of the process consists of giving the same participants an equal carbohydrate portion of the glucose (used as the reference food) and measuring their blood glucose response over the next two hours.

The Glycemic Index value for the food is then calculated for each participant by using a simple formula (dividing the blood glucose response for the food by their blood glucose response for the glucose (reference food)). The final value of the Glycemic Index for the food is the average Glycemic Index value for the participants (over 10).

Carbohydrates with a low GI value (55 or less) are more slowly digested, absorbed, and metabolized and cause a smaller and slower rise in blood glucose and, therefore, usually, insulin levels.

Low glycemic diet or foods are associated with the reduced risk of chronic disease. Foods that have low glycemic index are known for their property to release glucose in the blood slowly and regularly. Conversely, Foods that have a high glycemic index are known for their property to release glucose rapidly. Researches suggest that foods with a low glycemic index (LGI foods) are ideal for weight loss diets and foster lasting weight loss, in addition to their positive effect on the pancreas (insulin release), eyes, and kidney.

Glycemic Load

Basing your food choices only on the GI means that you're focusing on only one aspect of the food and ignoring other important aspects, such as the quality and quantity of the carbohydrates in the foods. Here comes the importance of the glycemic load which combines the two criteria and provides when available an additional tool for a better weight loss control and effective diabetes management.

Glycemic Load was introduced later to fill the gap and represents another critical tool to track carbohydrates quality and quantity. Glycemic Load (GL) combines both the quality and amount of carbohydrates following a simple formula:

Glycemic Load (GL) = GI x Carbohydrate (grams) content per portion ÷ 100

For example, an apple that has a GI of 32 and contains 13 grams of carbohydrates is considered as more healthier than Sweet potato that has a GL of 11 using the glycemic load tool.

Like the glycemic index, the glycemic load (GL) of a food can be classified as:

- **Low:** 10 or less
- **Medium:** 11 – 19
- **High:** 20 or more

Limitations of the concept

The glycemic index & glycemic load are great tools, but they do have a few limitations that you need to know:

- The lists of GI are quite limited. G.I. testing is new, and the process is expensive, time and resource consuming.
- The glycemic index depends on some external intervention like cooking. Al Dente Pasta are known to have a Lower Glycemic Index
- The testing results may vary. Researchers rely on the observation of tests involving participants metabolism to measure glycemic index as explained

in the previous section. This explains why GI may vary from studies.

Despite these limitations, the glycemic index & glycemic load are very useful tools that will help you achieve your goals in term of weight loss, health and disease prevention.

Chapter 1

THE GLYCEMIC DIET FOR
WEIGHT LOSS

IF YOU SEARCH FOR LOW-GI DIETS ONLINE, YOU'LL FIND A LOT OF promising weight-loss miracles along without any evidence-based science or related research. If you decide to go further and try to implement such methods, you will be sure to run into flaws and inconsistencies because the GI diet unlike many other diets didn't provide formal guidelines, nor provide optimal daily foods intake as many claims.

By keeping in mind that the glycemic index diet is rather an eating plan or a lifestyle, will increase your awareness on how to achieve a lasting weight loss, or maintain a healthy condition by eating according to the glycemic index.

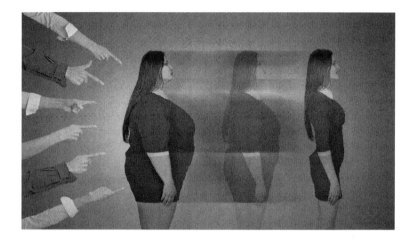

Fortunately, the science behind weight loss is today better developed especially the link between hormones and weight gain and obesity. Therefore, if you want to lose weight you have to understand how some specific hormones are involved in the weight gain process and how to make them work for you just by eating good carbohydrates (low-GI foods).

THIS CHAPTER WILL DISCUSS the legitimate science behind weight gain, satiety, anger, and hormones and shows you how incorporating low-GI foods into your daily intakes is the masterpiece of the weight-loss process, because those high-quality foods will help to minimize cravings, to reduce the risk of insulin resistance and to suppress your appetite.

Hormones That Regulate Body Weight

1- The Insulin hormone

Insulin is a polypeptide hormone that regulates the absorption of sugar by body cells and maintains the level of sugar present in the blood at a healthy level.. This hormone is produced by the β cells of the pancreas. When we eat, food travels to our stomach and intestines where it is broken down into micronutrients. These micronutrients are absorbed and transported by our bloodstream. The pancreas, which is the main regulator of our blood sugar, produces the insulin hormone, and releases it into the bloodstream when we eat. Insulin is a hormone that controls the level of glucose in the blood by controlling its production by the liver and its use by the muscle. Its primary function is to allow body cells, including muscles and other cells to absorb and transform sugar (glucose) into energy throughout the body.

Insulin sends also signals to liver, muscle, and adipocytes (fat cells) to store the excess of glucose for further use. Excess sugar is stored in 3 ways:

• In muscle tissues in the form of glycogen.

• In the liver in the form of glycogen.

• In adipose tissue (fat reserves of the body) in the form of triglycerides which are fat molecules that store energy

Weight gain and insulin

Weight gain is explained by the secretion of insulin. Insulin is the hormone responsible for weight gain secreted by the pancreas. If you do not secrete pancreas insulin, you do not gain weight.

Hyperglycemia is the abnormally high blood sugar level. Hyperglycemia is felt like a rush of adrenaline, a gain of energy, making us feel extremely good.

However, hyperglycemia lasts only a short time because when the blood sugar level is too high, the pancreas will secrete insulin to release the sugar in the blood and pass it to the cells.

As seen earlier, excess of sugar is stored in 3 ways, including in adipose tissue (fat reserves of the body) in the form of triglycerides which are fat molecules that store energy.

Refined sugar and starches consumption have also been associated with a higher risk of obesity, insulin resistance, fatty liver, metabolic syndrome, and a higher risk of chronic disease.

Insulin Resistance

Insulin resistance is a serious and silent health condition that occurs when cells in your muscles, liver and body fat start ignoring the signal that insulin hormone is sending out in order to transfer sugar (glucose) out of the bloodstream and put it into your body cells.

As insulin resistance develops, the body reacts by producing more and more insulin to lower the blood sugar.

Over time (months or years depending on the severity of the metabolic disfunction), the β cells in the pancreas that are working hard to make a higher supply of insulin, can no longer keep working to provide more and more insulin. Consequently, your blood sugar may reflect the pancreas failure to maintain the level in the healthy range, and your blood sugar begins to rise, indicating pre-diabetes or at worst diabetes type 2.

Symptoms of insulin resistance

Insulin resistance is silent and presents no symptoms in the first stage of its development. The symptoms start to appear later when the condition worsens, and the pancreas fails to produce enough amount of insulin to keep your blood sugar within the normal ranges. When this occurs, the symptoms may include:

- Excessive hunger Lethargy or tiredness Difficulty concentrating Brain fog
- Waist weight gain

• High blood pressure

Can insulin resistance be reduced or reversed?

Fortunately, It is possible to reduce the effects of insulin resistance and boost your insulin sensitivity by following a number of effective methods, including:

• Low glycemic diet
• Low carbohydrate and high-fat diet
• Low-calorie diets
• Weight loss surgery
• Regular exercise in combination with healthy diets

These methods have a similar way of working in that they all reduce the daily glucose intake drastically, lower the body's need for insulin, reduce insulin spike in the bloodstream, promote weight loss and prevent weight gain.

* * *

2- THE CORTISOL HORMONE

CORTISOL IS THE STRESS HORMONE, produced by the adrenal gland when the body is in stressful situations. The hypothalamus, via the pituitary gland, sends a chemical signal to the adrenal glands to produce and release both adrenaline and cortisol.

Cortisol is naturally released every day in small and regular quantities. However, like adrenaline, cortisol can also be secreted and released in reaction to physical and emotional stress and triggers the body's fight-or-flight response.

These two stress hormones work simultaneously: adrenaline produces a significant increase in strength, performance, awareness, and increases metabolism. It also let fat cells to release additional energy. Cortisol helps the body produce glucose from proteins, and increase the body's energy in times of stress quickly.

However, cortisol is also involved in a variety of essential function for your health. Most of the body cells have cortisol receptors to use this steroid hormone for a variety of critical functions, including:
- blood sugar regulation
- metabolism regulation
- inflammation reduction
- memory formulation

Cortisol is important for your health, but an excess of cortisol can harm your body and induce a variety of unwanted symptoms.

What cause high cortisol levels?

A high cortisol level can be caused by several things. High cortisol is known as Cushing syndrome. This health condition results from your body secreting and releasing too much cortisol.

Cushing syndrome causes many unwanted symptoms, including:

- obesity
- weight gain
- fatty deposits, especially in the face, midsection, and between the shoulders
- purple stretch marks on the arms, breasts, thighs, and abdomen
- thinning skin
- slow-healing injuries

Being under stress, induce a constant state of excess cortisol production. And, as seen above, this cortisol drives excess glucose production in a non-fight-or-flight situation. This excess glucose is converted into fat and stored by the body.

Thus, high levels of produced cortisol increase the risk of obesity highly, induce abdominal obesity, and increased the amount of fat storage.

Other factors that cause peaks in cortisol production are carbohydrates deprivation (in low carb diet, for example) and overconsumption of simple carbohydrates.

In both cases, when blood sugar levels fall, this induces a surge of stress hormones, including cortisol and adrenaline.

Stress hormones and their role in the body

Stress hormones are released in reply to body stressors. Hormonal responses of the woman body to stress are essential provided they occur in less frequently. They may become damaging and unhealthy when they happen too often. Prolonged exposure to porn induce severe damages to the brain and presents evidence that porn is not a healthy stressor.

Stress is habitually accompanied by high energy demand. Consequently, a severe stress situation induces a fast glucose release into the blood, which provides the required energy to deal with the stressful situation.

The principal players in the stress mechanism are: The adreno-corticotropic hormone (ACTH),

The glucocorticoids such as cortisol, adrenaline and nora-drenaline.

When this happens, blood glucose levels rise, concurrently with heart rate and blood pressure.

So at its simplest, stress leads to an increase in blood glucose, heart rate, and blood pressure, which induces an increased insulin release.

3- The Leptin Hormone

Leptin referred to as the starvation, or "hunger hormone" is an hormone produced by fat tissues and is secreted into our bloodstream. It plays an important role in weight regulation by reducing a person's appetite.

The Leptin hormone was discovered in 1994 and has gained significant interest for its powerful function in weight regulation and obesity. Leptin communicates with specific centers of the brain to influence how the body manages its store of fat. It sends a signal to the brain that the body has enough amount of stored fat, producing the body to burn calories from stored fat and reducing appetite.

Indeed, leptin plays the key regulator of body fat, and send signals to the brain to burn stored fat. This powerful effect would normally prevent obesity, overweight. Early researches have seen in leptin the solution for obesity. A supplementation of leptin would induce body fat burning, weight loss, and weight gain prevention. However, experiments revealed an unknown phenomenon which became until now, not fully understood.

Leptin resistance

Because leptin is produced by fat tissues, it is released in the bloodstream proportionally to the weight of a person. Its levels are high for people who are in overweight or obese than in people having normal weight.

However, researches have shown that the benefit of leptin in appetite-reducing is very low for obese people suggesting that people in obesity condition aren't sensitive to the beneficial effect of leptin and have developed Leptin resistance.

Leptin resistance is an abnormal condition that is associated with more weight gain for people in overweight or obesity.

Thus, obese people tend to eat more and more because the hormonal signal that normally send to the brain that the body has enough amount of stored fat seems to be ignored.

Ongoing researches are focusing on this kind of leptin resistance in obese people which stops the brain acknowledging the leptin's signal. Some studies, however, suggest that obesity induces multiple cellular processes that attenuate or prevent leptin signaling, amplifying the extent of weight gain. Leptin Resistance may arise from poor leptin transport across the blood-brain barrier (BBB), alteration of the leptin receptor, and defect of leptin signaling...

Ways to Improve Leptin Resistance and Promote Weight Loss

Strong evidence shows that Leptin resistance can be drastically reduced by following these guidelines:

- Eat low-glycemic and moderate-glycemic foods
- Avoid Ultra-processed food: the impact of Ultra-processed food is still under studies, but many pieces of evidence suggest that these kinds of foods compromise the integrity of your gut, the normal functioning and the production of gut hormones.
- Lower your triglycerides: Having high triglycerides level in your bloodstream can prevent the transport of leptin to your brain.
- Eat healthy protein: Eating healthy proteins can improve leptin sensitivity.
- Eat healthy fats and keep your ratio omega 6/ omega 3 inferior to 3.
- Avoid simple carbohydrates, starches, and eat healthy carbohydrates (complex carbs, fiber).

4- The Ghrelin Hormone

Ghrelin, known as the "hunger hormone," is an acyl-peptide responsible for stimulating hunger by sending a chemical signal to tells you when to eat. Ghrelin is secreted and released primarily by the stomach. Smaller amounts of this hormone are also secreted by the small intestine, and pancreas.

Ghrelin has various functions. It is known mainly as the hormone that triggers hunger by stimulating the appetite. It induces increases in food intake and promotes fat storage and weight gain.

These findings suggest that by controlling the level of gherkin and let it down, we can reduce appetite and food intake.

An experiment consisting of administering ghrelin to people concluded that food intake was increased by 30% in this population.

How is ghrelin controlled?

Ghrelin levels are mainly regulated by food intake. Levels of ghrelin in the bloodstream rise typically before eating and when fasting in line with increased hunger.

Experimental studies demonstrated that Ghrelin levels are lower in obese or overweight individuals. Conversely, lean individuals have a high level of ghrelin.

Studies also found that some foods (low-GI foods) slow down the ghrelin release in the bloodstream and thus reduce the impact of the hormones of hunger.

Soluble and insoluble fibers inhibit ghrelin secretion, which implies that eating complex carbohydrates (low-GI and moderate-GI foods) has a positive and significant effect in reducing the production and release of ghrelin.

Glucose also has the same effect as dietary fibers in inhibiting Ghrelin secretion. However, as seen earlier, glucose, starches, and simple carbohydrates must be prohibited due to their impact in rising insulin release.

Recent studies demonstrated that contrary to a common belief, proteins did not reduce the production or release of ghrelin.

5- The PYY family

The gut hormone peptide YY 3–36 (PYY3–36) is a polypeptide hormone released from L-cells found in large intestine and the intestinal mucosa of the ileum.

The hormone PYY is released proportionally to nutrient intake. Indeed, the amount of this hormone is strongly influenced by the number of calories consumed, the macronutrient and micronutrient composition of the eaten meal.

After eating, PYY levels rise within the fifteen first minutes and reach a peak level within ninety minutes. Its main role is to reduce appetite, the psychological driver for eating. It also plays an important role in regulating the energy balance in the body.

Higher levels of PYY results on reduced appetite and consequently reduced calorie intake, and help in weight loss.

Conversely, low levels of PYY induce strong feelings of hunger and cravings, while predisposing fatty tissue retention.

That implies that calorie intake matters, thus you have to restrict your daily intake to lose weight. You can calculate the calorie deficit you need to achieve your goal in term of weight loss by using our calculator online: https://www.easyketodiet. net/advanced-keto-calculator/

Your ideal daily calorie intake will be calculated taking into account several factors such as your gender, height, weight, metabolism, activity...

Chapter 2

LOW GLYCEMIC INDEX
FOODS TABLES

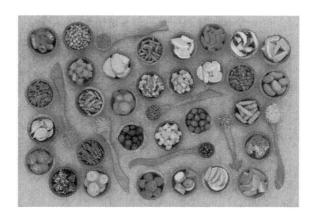

Low glycemic index (GI value of 55 or less): foods in this category must be included in a GI diet in the first intent since their effects on the blood sugar levels are moderate, they include most vegetables and fruits, beans, **low**-fat dairy **foods,** pasta, minimally processed grains, and nuts. PS. Cooking can influence the GI positively or negatively.

Food Name: 3 Grain Bread, sprouted grains
GI = 55
Serving (g): 30

GL = 5

Food Name: 45% oat bran and 50% wheat flour bread
GI = 50
Serving (g): 30
GL = 9

Food Name: 50% oat bran bread
GI = 44
Serving (g): 30
GL = 8

Food Name: 9-Grain Multi-Grain bread
GI = 43
Serving (g): 30
GL = 6

Food Name: American, easy-cook rice, consumed with 10 g
margarine
GI = 49
Serving (g): 150
GL = 22

Food Name: Apple and blackcurrant juice, no added sugar
GI = 45
Serving (g): 250
GL = 11

Food Name: Apple and cherry juice, pure, unsweetened
GI = 43
Serving (g): 250
GL = 14

Food Name: Apple and mango juice, pure, unsweetened
GI = 47

Serving (g): 250

GL = 16

Food Name: Apple blueberry muffin

GI = 49

Serving (g): 60

GL = 12

Food Name: Apple juice, Granny Smith, unsweetened

GI = 44

Serving (g): 250

GL = 13

Food Name: Apple juice, pure, clear, unsweetened

GI = 44

Serving (g): 250

GL = 13

Food Name: Apple juice, pure, cloudy, unsweetened

GI = 37

Serving (g): 250

GL = 11

Food Name: Apple juice, unsweetened, reconstituted

GI = 39

Serving (g): 250

GL = 10

Food Name: Apple muffin, made with rolled oats and
sugar

GI = 44

Serving (g): 60

GL = 13

Food Name: Apple muffin, made with rolled oats and without
sugar
GI = 48
Serving (g): 60
GL = 9

Food Name: Apple, raw
GI = 36 ± 4
Serving (g): 120
GL = 5

Food Name: Apple, raw, Golden Delicious
GI = 39 ± 2
Serving (g): 120
GL = 6

Food Name: Apricot & apple fruit strips, gluten-free
GI = 29 ± 4
Serving (g): 20
GL = 5

Food Name: Apricot 100% Pure Fruit spread, no added sugar
GI = 43 ± 3
Serving (g): 30
GL = 7

Food Name: Apricot dried fruit snack
GI = 42 ± 4
Serving (g): 15
GL = 5

Food Name: Apricot fruit spread, reduced sugar
GI = 55 ± 2
Serving (g): 30

GL = 7

Food Name: Apricot halves canned in fruit juice
GI = 51 ± 4
Serving (g): 120
GL = 6

Food Name: Apricot, raw
GI = 34 ± 2
Serving (g): 120
GL = 3

Food Name: Apricots, dried
GI = 30 ± 2
Serving (g): 60
GL = 8

Food Name: Arepa, made from white corn meal flour
GI = 53 ± 2
Serving (g): 100
GL = 19

Food Name: Aussie Bodies Start the Day UHT, Choc Banana
flavored drink
GI = 24 ± 3
Serving (g): 250
GL = 4

Food Name: Aussie Bodies Start the Day UHT, Chocolate
flavored drink
GI = 26 ± 3
Serving (g): 250
GL = 4

Food Name: Aussie Bodies Trim Protein Shake, Chocolate
flavoured beverage
GI = 39 ± 3
Serving (g): 250
GL = 5

Food Name: Aussie Bodies Trim Protein Shake, French Vanilla
flavoured beverage
GI = 41 ± 2
Serving (g): 250
GL = 5

Food Name: Bakers Delight™ Hi Fibre Lo GI white bread
GI = 52 ± 2
Serving (g): 30
GL = 8

Food Name: Bakers Delight™ Wholemeal Country Grain bread
GI = 53 ± 2
Serving (g): 30
GL = 6

Food Name: Banana cake, made with sugar
GI = 47 ± 2
Serving (g): 60
GL = 14

Food Name: Banana cake, made without sugar
GI = 55 ± 2
Serving (g): 60
GL = 12

Food Name: Banana, over-ripe
GI = 52 ± 2

Serving (g): 120
GL = 11

Food Name: Banana, over-ripe (yellow flecked with brown)
GI = 48 ± 3
Serving (g): 120
GL = 12

Food Name: Banana, raw
GI = 47 ± 2
Serving (g): 120
GL = 11

Food Name: Banana, ripe (all yellow)
GI = 51 ± 2
Serving (g): 120
GL = 13

Food Name: Banana, slightly under-ripe (yellow with green sections)
GI = 42 ± 2
Serving (g): 120
GL = 11

Food Name: Banana, under-ripe
GI = 30 ± 2
Serving (g): 120
GL = 6

Food Name: Barley
GI = 23 ± 4
Serving (g): 150
GL = 11

Food Name: Barley kernels, high-amylose (covered), boiled in water for 25 min (kernel:water = 1:2)
GI = 26 ± 2
Serving (g): 150
GL = 11

Food Name: Barley kernels, high-amylose (hull-less) boiled in water for 25 min
GI = 20 ± 2
Serving (g): 150
GL = 8

Food Name: Barley kernels, waxy (hull-less), boiled in water for 25 min
GI = 22 ± 3
Serving (g): 150
GL = 9

Food Name: Barley, cracked (Malthouth, Tunisia)
GI = 50 ± 2
Serving (g): 150
GL = 21

Food Name: Barley, pearled
GI = 22 ± 3
Serving (g): 150
GL = 9

Food Name: Barley, pearled
GI = 29 ± 3
Serving (g): 150
GL = 12

Food Name: Barley, pearled, boiled 60 min

GI = 35 ± 2
Serving (g): 150
GL = 15

Food Name: Basmati, white rice, boiled 12 min
GI = 52 ± 2
Serving (g): 150
GL = 15

Food Name: Basmati, white rice, boiled, with 10 g margarine
GI = 43 ± 2
Serving (g): 150
GL = 18

Food Name: Blueberry muffin
GI = 50 ± 2
Serving (g): 60
GL = 15

Food Name: Breakfast Marmalade 100% Fruit Spread, Cottees™
brand
GI = 55 ± 3
Serving (g): 30
GL = 10

Food Name: Brown & Wild rice, Uncle Ben's® Ready Whole
Grain Medley™ (pouch)
GI = 45 ± 3
Serving (g): 150
GL = 18

Food Name: Brown & Wild rice, Uncle Ben's® Ready Whole
Grain Medley™ (pouch)
GI = 45 ± 2

Serving (g): 150
GL = 18

Food Name: Brown rice, steamed
GI = 50 ± 1
Serving (g): 150
GL = 16

Food Name: Brown Rice, Uncle Ben's® Ready Whole Grain (pouch)
GI = 48 ± 2
Serving (g): 150
GL = 20

Food Name: Buckwheat groats, hydrothermally treated, dehusked, boiled 12 min
GI = 45 ± 3
Serving (g): 150
GL = 13

Food Name: Buckwheat noodles, instant
GI = 53 ± 2
Serving (g): 180
GL = 22

Food Name: Build-Up™ nutrient-fortified drink, vanilla with fibre
GI = 41 ± 3
Serving (g): 250
GL = 13

Food Name: Butternut pumpkin, boiled
GI = 51 ± 2
Serving (g): 80

GL = 3

Food Name: Capellini pasta
GI = 45 ± 3
Serving (g): 180
GL = 20

Food Name: Capilano Premium Honey, blend of eucalypt &
floral honeys
GI = 51 ± 2
Serving (g): 25
GL = 11

Food Name: Carrot cake, prepared with coconut flour
GI = 36 ± 2
Serving (g): 60
GL = 8

Food Name: Carrot juice, freshly made
GI = 43 ± 2
Serving (g): 250
GL = 10

Food Name: Carrot soup, President's Choice® Blue Menu™
Soupreme
GI = 35 ± 3
Serving (g): 250
GL = 5

Food Name: Carrots, peeled, boiled
GI = 33 ± 2
Serving (g): 80
GL = 2

Food Name: Carrots, raw, diced
GI = 35 ± 2
Serving (g): 80
GL = 2

Food Name: Carrots, raw, ground
GI = 39 ± 4
Serving (g): 80
GL = 2

Food Name: Cashew nut halves
GI = 27 ± 2
Serving (g): 50
GL = 3

Food Name: Cashew nuts
GI = 25 ± 2
Serving (g): 50
GL = 3

Food Name: Cashew nuts, organic, roasted and salted
GI = 25 ± 2
Serving (g): 50
GL = 3

Food Name: Cashew nuts, roasted and salted
GI = 27 ± 2
Serving (g): 50
GL = 3

Food Name: Cereal bar, cranberry flavor
GI = 42 ± 3
Serving (g): 30
GL = 6

Food Name: Cereal bar, hazelnut flavor
GI = 33 ± 3
Serving (g): 30
GL = 4

Food Name: Cereal bar, orange flavor
GI = 33 ± 3
Serving (g): 30
GL = 5

Food Name: Cereal biscuit (30 g), cocoa flavor wheat biscuits
consumed with 125 mL skim milk
GI = 46 ± 3
Serving (g): 155
GL = 12

Food Name: Cereal biscuit (30 g), honey flavor wheat biscuits
consumed with 125 mL skim milk
GI = 52 ± 3
Serving (g): 155
GL = 14

Food Name: Cereal biscuit (30 g), wheat based biscuits
consumed with 125 mL skim milk
GI = 47 ± 3
Serving (g): 155
GL = 12

Food Name: Cherries, raw, sour
GI = 22 ± 2
Serving (g): 120
GL = 3

Food Name: Chicken Flavored Brown Rice, Uncle Ben's® Ready Whole Grain (pouch)
GI = 46 ± 3
Serving (g): 150
GL = 18

Food Name: Chicken Flavored Brown Rice, Uncle Ben's® Ready Whole Grain (pouch)
GI = 46 ± 3
Serving (g): 150
GL = 18

Food Name: Chicken McNuggets™ consumed with sweet Thai chilli sauce
GI = 55 ± 3
Serving (g): 100
GL = 12

Food Name: Chicken nuggets, frozen, reheated in microwave oven 5 min
GI = 46 ± 3
Serving (g): 100
GL = 7

Food Name: Chicken tikka masala and rice, convenience meal
GI = 34 ± 3
Serving (g): 300
GL = 21

Food Name: Chilli beef noodles, prepared convenience meal
GI = 42 ± 3
Serving (g): 300
GL = 19

Food Name: Chilli con carne, made from haricot beans
GI = 34 ± 3
Serving (g): 300
GL = 12

Food Name: Chocolate butterscotch muffin
GI = 53 ± 2
Serving (g): 50
GL = 15

Food Name: Chocolate cake made from packet mix with
chocolate frosting
GI = 38 ± 3
Serving (g): 111
GL = 20

Food Name: Chocolate candy, sugar free, artificially sweetened,
Dove®
GI = 23 ± 2
Serving (g): 50
GL = 3

Food Name: Chocolate chip muffin
GI = 52 ± 3
Serving (g): 60
GL = 17

Food Name: Chocolate crinkles, containing coconut flour
GI = 43 ± 3
Serving (g): 50
GL = 10

Food Name: Chocolate Daydream™ shake, fructose, Revival
Soy®

GI = 33 ± 3
Serving (g): 250
GL = 6

Food Name: Chocolate Daydream™ shake, sucralose, Revival Soy®
GI = 25 ± 3
Serving (g): 250
GL = 1

Food Name: Chocolate pudding, instant, made from powder and whole milk
GI = 47 ± 2
Serving (g): 100
GL = 7

Food Name: Chocolate, dark with raisins, peanuts and jam
GI = 44 ± 3
Serving (g): 50
GL = 12

Food Name: Chocolate, dark, Dove®
GI = 23 ± 4
Serving (g): 50
GL = 6

Food Name: Chocolate, plain
GI = 42 ± 4
Serving (g): 50
GL = 13

Food Name: Chocolate, plain with sucrose
GI = 34 ± 3
Serving (g): 50

GL = 7

Food Name: Citrus, reduced-fat mousse, prepared from commercial mousse mix with water
GI = 47 ± 2
Serving (g): 50
GL = 14

Food Name: Coarse rye kernel bread, 80% intact kernels and 20% white wheat flour
GI = 41 ± 3
Serving (g): 30
GL = 5

Food Name: Coarse wheat kernel bread, 80% intact kernels and 20% white wheat flour
GI = 52 ± 2
Serving (g): 30
GL = 10

Food Name: Cocoavia™ Chocolate Covered Almonds, artificially sweetened
GI = 21 ± 3
Serving (g): 30
GL = 2

Food Name: Coconut sugar
GI = 54 ± 1
Serving (g): 5
GL = 3

Food Name: Continental fruit loaf, wheat bread with dried fruit
GI = 47 ± 2

Serving (g): 30
GL = 7

Food Name: Corn granules
GI = 52 ± 1
Serving (g): 150
GL = 15

Food Name: Corn tortilla
GI = 52 ± 1
Serving (g): 50
GL = 12

Food Name: Corn tortilla, made from white corn, Diego's brand
GI = 49 ± 3
Serving (g): 50
GL = 11

Food Name: Corn tortilla, served with refried mashed pinto beans and tomato sauce
GI = 39 ± 2
Serving (g): 100
GL = 9

Food Name: Country Grain Organic Rye bread
GI = 53 ± 2
Serving (g): 30
GL = 5

Food Name: Cranberry & Orange Soy muffin, President's Choice® Blue Menu™
GI = 48 ± 2
Serving (g): 70
GL = 14

Food Name: Cranberry juice cocktail
GI = 52 ± 1
Serving (g): 250
GL = 16

Food Name: Crème fraiche dessert, peach
GI = 28 ± 1
Serving (g): 150
GL = 7

Food Name: Crème fraiche dessert, raspberry
GI = 30 ± 1
Serving (g): 150
GL = 5

Food Name: Crusty malted wheat bread
GI = 52 ± 1
Serving (g): 30
GL = 7

Food Name: Double chocolate muffin
GI = 46 ± 2
Serving (g): 60
GL = 16

Food Name: English Muffin bread, Whole Grain Multigrain,
President's Choice® Blue Menu™
GI = 45 ± 3
Serving (g): 30
GL = 5

Food Name: Fettucine, egg
GI = 32 ± 1
Serving (g): 180

GL = 15

Food Name: Fish fingers
GI = 38 ± 1
Serving (g): 100
GL = 7

Food Name: Fromage Frais, red fruit: blackcurrant
GI = 22 ± 1
Serving (g): 100
GL = 2

Food Name: Fromage Frais, red fruit: raspberry
GI = 31 ± 1
Serving (g): 100
GL = 2

Food Name: Fromage Frais, red fruit: red cherry
GI = 25 ± 1
Serving (g): 100
GL = 2

Food Name: Fructose, 25 g portion, Sweeten Less
GI = 11
Serving (g): 10
GL = 1

Food Name: Fructose, 50 g portion
GI = 20
Serving (g): 10
GL = 2

Food Name: Fructose, 50 g portion
GI = 23

Serving (g): 10
GL = 2

Food Name: Fructose, 50 g portion, Sweeten Less
GI = 12
Serving (g): 10
GL = 1

Food Name: Fruit and Spice Loaf bread, thick sliced
GI = 54 ± 1
Serving (g): 30
GL = 8

Food Name: Fusilli pasta twists, boiled 10 min in salted water,
served with cheddar cheese
GI = 27 ± 2
Serving (g): 0
GL = 0

Food Name: Fusilli pasta twists, boiled 10 min in salted water,
served with canned tuna
GI = 28 ± 2
Serving (g): 0
GL = 0

Food Name: Fusilli pasta twists, boiled 10 min in salted water,
served with chilli con carne
GI = 40 ± 3
Serving (g): 0
GL = 0

Food Name: Fusilli pasta twists, dry pasta, boiled in 10 min in
unsalted water
GI = 54 ± 1

Serving (g): 180

GL = 26

Food Name: Fusilli pasta twists, tricolour, dry pasta, boiled 10 min in unsalted water

GI = 51 ± 1

Serving (g): 180

GL = 23

Food Name: Fusilli pasta twists, wholewheat, dry pasta, boiled 10 min in unsalted water

GI = 55 ± 1

Serving (g): 180

GL = 23

Food Name: Gluten Free Low GI White bread

GI = 53

Serving (g): 30

GL = 4

Food Name: Gluten-free pasta, maize starch, boiled 8 min

GI = 54 ± 1

Serving (g): 180

GL = 23

Food Name: Gluten-free pasta, maize starch, boiled 8 min

GI = 54 ± 1

Serving (g): 180

GL = 23

Food Name: Golden Hearth™ Organic Heavy Wholegrain bread

GI = 53 ± 1

Serving (g): 30

GL = 7

Food Name: Grapefruit, raw
GI = 25 ± 2
Serving (g): 120
GL = 3

Food Name: Grapefruit, ruby red segments, canned in juice
GI = 47 ± 2
Serving (g): 120
GL = 10

Food Name: Grapes, raw
GI = 45 ± 4
Serving (g): 120
GL = 7

Food Name: Green banana, peeled, boiled 10 min
GI = 37 ± 2
Serving (g): 120
GL = 10

Food Name: Ground beef served with rice and an orange
GI = 31 ± 2
Serving (g): 300
GL = 24

Food Name: Haricot beans, home-cooked, soaked overnight, boiled 1h in water, baked in tomato sauce 2h
GI = 23 ± 2
Serving (g): 150
GL = 7

Food Name: Haricot/Navy beans

GI = 39 ± 2
Serving (g): 150
GL = 12

Food Name: Haricot/Navy beans, boiled
GI = 31 ± 2
Serving (g): 150
GL = 9

Food Name: Hazelnut, 2.4% fat mousse, prepared from commercial mousse mix with water
GI = 36 ± 2
Serving (g): 50
GL = 4

Food Name: Healthy Choice™ Hearty 7 Grain bread
GI = 55 ± 1
Serving (g): 30
GL = 8

Food Name: Honey Crunch cereal (30 g), consumed with 125 mL skim milk
GI = 54 ± 2
Serving (g): 155
GL = 16

Food Name: Honey, Iron Bark (34% fructose)
GI = 48 ± 1
Serving (g): 25
GL = 7

Food Name: Honey, Red Gum (35% fructose)
GI = 46 ± 1
Serving (g): 25

GL = 8

Food Name: Honey, Stringy Bark (52% fructose)
GI = 44 ± 1
Serving (g): 25
GL = 9

Food Name: Honey, Yapunya (42 % fructose)
GI = 52 ± 1
Serving (g): 25
GL = 9

Food Name: Honey, Yellow box (46% fructose)
GI = 35 ± 1
Serving (g): 25
GL = 6

Food Name: Hot oat cereal (30 g) prepared with 125 mL
skim milk
GI = 47 ± 1
Serving (g): 155
GL = 11

Food Name: Hot oat cereal (30 g), berry flavor prepared with 125
mL skim milk
GI = 43 ± 1
Serving (g): 155
GL = 11

Food Name: Hot oat cereal (30 g), cocoa flavor prepared with 125
mL skim milk
GI = 40 ± 1
Serving (g): 155
GL = 9

Food Name: Hot oat cereal (30 g), fruit flavor prepared with 125 mL skim milk
GI = 47 ± 1
Serving (g): 155
GL = 12

Food Name: Hot oat cereal (30 g), honey flavor prepared with 125 mL skim milk
GI = 47 ± 1
Serving (g): 155
GL = 12

Food Name: Hot oat cereal (30 g), orchard fruit flavor prepared with 125 mL skim milk
GI = 50 ± 1
Serving (g): 155
GL = 12

Food Name: Ice cream, low-fat, Bulla Light Creamy vanilla
GI = 36 ± 1
Serving (g): 50
GL = 7

Food Name: Ice cream, low-fat, Bulla Light Real Dairy chocolate
GI = 27 ± 1
Serving (g): 50
GL = 3

Food Name: Ice cream, low-fat, Bulla Light Real Dairy mango
GI = 30
Serving (g): 50
GL = 4

Food Name: Ice cream, low-fat, Light & Creamy, Raspberry
Ripple
GI = 55 ± 1
Serving (g): 50
GL = 9

Food Name: Ice cream, low-fat, vanilla, 'Light'
GI = 46 ± 2
Serving (g): 50
GL = 7

Food Name: Instant 'two-minute' noodles, Maggi® (Nestlé,
Auckland, New Zealand)
GI = 48 ± 2
Serving (g): 180
GL = 12

Food Name: Instant 'two-minute' noodles, Maggi® (Nestlé,
Australia) (1995)
GI = 46 ± 2
Serving (g): 180
GL = 11

Food Name: Instant 'two-minute' noodles, Maggi®, all flavors
(Nestlé Australia) (2005)
GI = 52 ± 2
Serving (g): 180
GL = 13

Food Name: Instant noodles, all flavors (Woolworths Limited,
Australia)
GI = 52 ± 2
Serving (g): 180
GL = 11

Food Name: Instant rice, white, cooked 3 min
GI = 46 ± 3
Serving (g): 150
GL = 19

Food Name: Kidney beans
GI = 29 ± 2
Serving (g): 150
GL = 7

Food Name: Kiwi fruit, Hayward
GI = 47 ± 2
Serving (g): 120
GL = 6

Food Name: Lasagne sheets, dry pasta, boiled in unsalted water
for 10 min
GI = 55 ± 2
Serving (g): 180
GL = 26

Food Name: Lasagne, egg, dry pasta, boiled in unsalted water
for 10 min
GI = 53 ± 2
Serving (g): 180
GL = 23

Food Name: Lasagne, egg, verdi, dry pasta, boiled in unsalted
water for 10 min
GI = 52 ± 2
Serving (g): 180
GL = 23

Food Name: Lemonade, Scheweppes®, lemon soft drink

GI = 54 ± 4
Serving (g): 250
GL = 15

Food Name: Lentils, brown, canned, drained, Edgell's™ brand
GI = 42 ± 2
Serving (g): 150
GL = 9

Food Name: Lentils, green, dried, boiled
GI = 37 ± 2
Serving (g): 150
GL = 5

Food Name: Lentils, red, split, dried, boiled 25 min
GI = 21 ± 2
Serving (g): 150
GL = 4

Food Name: Lentils, raw
GI = 29 ± 2
Serving (g): 150
GL = 5

Food Name: Long Grain and Wild, Jasmine rice, Uncle Ben's®
Ready Rice (pouch)
GI = 49 ± 3
Serving (g): 150
GL = 21

Food Name: Long Grain and Wild, Jasmine rice, Uncle Ben's®
Ready Rice (pouch)
GI = 49 ± 3
Serving (g): 150

GL = 21

Food Name: Long grain rice quick-cooking variety, white, pre-
cooked, microwaved 2 min, Express Rice, plain
GI = 52 ± 3
Serving (g): 150
GL = 19

Food Name: Long grain rice quick-cooking variety, white, pre-
cooked, microwaved 2 min, Express Rice, plain
GI = 52 ± 3
Serving (g): 150
GL = 19

Food Name: Low-fat yoghurt, apricot
GI = 42 ± 1
Serving (g): 200
GL = 12

Food Name: Low-fat yoghurt, black cherry
GI = 41 ± 1
Serving (g): 200
GL = 11

Food Name: Low-fat yoghurt, hazelnut
GI = 53 ± 1
Serving (g): 200
GL = 15

Food Name: Low-fat yoghurt, Nestlé Diet Mixed Berry
GI = 28 ± 1
Serving (g): 200
GL = 3

Food Name: Low-fat yoghurt, Nestlé Diet Peaches & Cream
GI = 28 ± 1
Serving (g): 200
GL = 3

Food Name: Low-fat yoghurt, raspberry
GI = 34 ± 1
Serving (g): 200
GL = 10

Food Name: LU P'tit Déjeuner Chocolat cookies
GI = 42 ± 3
Serving (g): 50
GL = 14

Food Name: LU P'tit Déjeuner Miel et Pépites Chocolat cookies
GI = 45 ± 3
Serving (g): 50
GL = 16

Food Name: LU P'tit Déjeuner Miel et Pépites Chocolat cookies
GI = 49 ± 3
Serving (g): 50
GL = 18

Food Name: LU P'tit Déjeuner Miel et Pépites Chocolat cookies
GI = 52 ± 3
Serving (g): 50
GL = 18

Food Name: LU Petit Dejeuner Cereals & Chocolate Chips, low
in sugar cookies
GI = 37 ± 3
Serving (g): 50

GL = 13

Food Name: LU Petit Dejeuner Chocolate & Cereals cookies
GI = 46 ± 3
Serving (g): 50
GL = 16

Food Name: LU Petit Dejeuner Coconut, nuts and chocolate
cookies
GI = 51 ± 3
Serving (g): 50
GL = 17

Food Name: LU Petit Dejeuner Coconut, nuts and chocolate
cookies
GI = 55 ± 3
Serving (g): 50
GL = 19

Food Name: LU Petit Dejeuner Fruits and Muesli cookies
GI = 45 ± 3
Serving (g): 50
GL = 16

Food Name: LU Petit Dejeuner Fruits and Muesli cookies
GI = 47 ± 3
Serving (g): 50
GL = 17

Food Name: LU Petit Dejeuner Fruits and Muesli cookies
GI = 49 ± 3
Serving (g): 50
GL = 18

Food Name: LU Petit Dejeuner Honey & Chocolate chips
cookies
GI = 46 ± 3
Serving (g): 50
GL = 16

Food Name: LU Petit Dejeuner Honey & Chocolate chips
cookies
GI = 47 ± 3
Serving (g): 50
GL = 17

Food Name: LU Petit Dejeuner Milk and Cereals cookies
GI = 39 ± 3
Serving (g): 50
GL = 13

Food Name: LU Petit Dejeuner Milk and Cereals cookies
GI = 55 ± 3
Serving (g): 50
GL = 19

Food Name: LU Petit Dejeuner Multicereals cookies
GI = 46 ± 3
Serving (g): 50
GL = 16

Food Name: LU Petit Dejeuner with Fruits and Figs cookies
GI = 41 ± 3
Serving (g): 50
GL = 14

Food Name: LU Petit Dejeuner with Prunes cookies
GI = 51 ± 3

Serving (g): 50
GL = 17

Food Name: LU Petit Dejeuner, Chocolate, low in sugar cookies
GI = 51 ± 3
Serving (g): 50
GL = 18

Food Name: Mandarin segments, canned in juice
GI = 47 ± 2
Serving (g): 120
GL = 6

Food Name: Mango, raw
GI = 41 ± 2
Serving (g): 120
GL = 8

Food Name: Mango, 1.8% fat mousse, prepared from
commercial mousse mix with water
GI = 33 ± 2
Serving (g): 50
GL = 4

Food Name: Mango, low-fat frozen fruit dessert, Frutia™
GI = 42 ± 2
Serving (g): 100
GL = 10

Food Name: Marmalade, orange
GI = 48 ± 2
Serving (g): 30
GL = 9

Food Name: Marmalade, orange 100% Pure Fruit spread, no added sugar
GI = 27 ± 2
Serving (g): 30
GL = 4

Food Name: Mars Active® Energy Drink, flavored milk
GI = 46 ± 3
Serving (g): 250
GL = 15

Food Name: Milk, full-fat/whole
GI = 36 ± 4
Serving (g): 250
GL = 4

Food Name: Milk, reduced fat
GI = 30 ± 4
Serving (g): 250
GL = 4

Food Name: Milk, semi-skimmed
GI = 32 ± 2
Serving (g): 250
GL = 4

Food Name: Milk, skim
GI = 32 ± 2
Serving (g): 250
GL = 4

Food Name: Mixed berry, 2.2% fat mousse, prepared from commercial mousse mix with water
GI = 36 ± 2

Serving (g): 50
GL = 4

Food Name: Mixed nuts and raisins
GI = 21 ± 2
Serving (g): 50
GL = 3

Food Name: Mixed nuts, roasted and salted
GI = 24 ± 2
Serving (g): 50
GL = 4

Food Name: Moolgiri white rice
GI = 54 ± 2
Serving (g): 150
GL = 17

Food Name: Muesli, gluten-free with 1.5% fat milk (125 mL)
GI = 39 ± 2
Serving (g): 30
GL = 7

Food Name: Muesli, toasted
GI = 43 ± 2
Serving (g): 30
GL = 7

Food Name: Muesli, Wheat free, consumed with 150 mL semi-
skimmed milk
GI = 49 ± 2
Serving (g): 30
GL = 9

Food Name: Muesli, yeast & wheat free
GI = 45 ± 2
Serving (g): 30
GL = 4

Food Name: Muffin, plain, made from wheat flour
GI = 46 ± 2
Serving (g): 50
GL = 11

Food Name: Muffin, reduced-fat, low-calorie, made from high-amylose corn starch and maltitol
GI = 37 ± 3
Serving (g): 50
GL = 9

Food Name: Multigrain (50% kibbled wheat grain) bread
GI = 43 ± 2
Serving (g): 30
GL = 6

Food Name: Multigrain Loaf bread, spelt wheat flour
GI = 54 ± 2
Serving (g): 30
GL = 8

Food Name: Multigrain porridge, containing rolled oats, wheat, triticale, rye, barley and rice, cooked with water
GI = 55 ± 2
Serving (g): 250
GL = 19

Food Name: Multiseed bread
GI = 54 ± 2

Serving (g): 30
GL = 7

Food Name: Nectarines, raw
GI = 43 ± 2
Serving (g): 120
GL = 4

Food Name: Oat porridge made from roasted thick (1.0 mm)
GI = 50 ± 1
Serving (g): 250
GL = 14

Food Name: Oat porridge made from steamed thick (1.0 mm)
dehulled oat flakes
GI = 53 ± 1
Serving (g): 250
GL = 14

Food Name: Orange & Grapefruit segments, canned in juice
GI = 53 ± 2
Serving (g): 120
GL = 10

Food Name: Orange Delight Cocktail beverage with pulp,
President's Choice® Blue Menu™
GI = 44 ± 2
Serving (g): 250
GL = 7
Food Name: Orange juice
GI = 46 ± 2
Serving (g): 250
GL = 12

Food Name: Orange juice, unsweetened, reconstituted
concentrate, Commercial brand
GI = 54 ± 2
Serving (g): 250
GL = 11

Food Name: Orange, raw
GI = 38 ± 7
Serving (g): 120
GL = 7

Food Name: Original Long Grain, Jasmine rice, Uncle Ben's®
Ready Rice (pouch)
GI = 48 ± 3
Serving (g): 150
GL = 22

Food Name: Original Long Grain, Jasmine rice, Uncle Ben's®
Ready Rice (pouch)
GI = 48 ± 3
Serving (g): 150
GL = 22

Food Name: Pancakes, prepared with coconut flour
GI = 46 ± 3
Serving (g): 80
GL = 10

Food Name: Pasta bake, tomato and mozzarella
GI = 23 ± 3
Serving (g): 300
GL = 10

Food Name: Peach & Grapes, canned in natural fruit juice

GI = 46 ± 2
Serving (g): 120
GL = 6

Food Name: Peach & pear fruit strips, gluten-free
GI = 29 ± 2
Serving (g): 20
GL = 3

Food Name: Peach & Pineapple, canned in natural fruit juice
GI = 45 ± 2
Serving (g): 120
GL = 6

Food Name: Peach, canned in light syrup
GI = 52 ± 2
Serving (g): 120
GL = 9

Food Name: Peach, canned in natural juice
GI = 45 ± 2
Serving (g): 120
GL = 5

Food Name: Peach, dried
GI = 35 ± 2
Serving (g): 60
GL = 8

Food Name: Peach, raw
GI = 28 ± 2
Serving (g): 120
GL = 4

Food Name: Peanuts, crushed
GI = 7 ± 2
Serving (g): 50
GL = 0

Food Name: Pear halves, canned in natural juice
GI = 43 ± 2
Serving (g): 120
GL = 5

Food Name: Pear, dried
GI = 43 ± 2
Serving (g): 60
GL = 12

Food Name: Pear, raw
GI = 33 ± 4
Serving (g): 120
GL = 4

Food Name: Pineapple, raw
GI = 51 ± 2
Serving (g): 120
GL = 8

Food Name: Pineapple & Papaya pieces, canned in natural juice
GI = 53 ± 2
Serving (g): 120
GL = 9

Food Name: Pineapple pieces, canned in natural fruit juice
GI = 55 ± 2
Serving (g): 120
GL = 10

Food Name: Ploughman's™ Wholegrain bread, original recipe
GI = 47 ± 2
Serving (g): 30
GL = 6

Food Name: Plum, raw
GI = 40 ± 2
Serving (g): 120
GL = 7

Food Name: Popcorn
GI = 55 ± 2
Serving (g): 20
GL = 6

Food Name: Porridge oats, made from rolled oats
GI = 50 ± 2
Serving (g): 250
GL = 10

Food Name: Porridge, jumbo oats, consumed with 150 mL semi-skimmed milk
GI = 40 ± 2
Serving (g): 250
GL = 9

Food Name: Porridge, made from rolled oats
GI = 55 ± 2
Serving (g): 250
GL = 13

Food Name: Potato crisps, plain, salted
GI = 51 ± 2
Serving (g): 50

GL = 12

Food Name: Pound cake
GI = 38 ± 2
Serving (g): 60
GL = 9

Food Name: Proti pasta, protein-enriched, boiled in water
GI = 28 ± 2
Serving (g): 180
GL = 14

Food Name: Prune juice
GI = 43 ± 2
Serving (g): 250
GL = 15

Food Name: Prunes, pitted
GI = 29 ± 2
Serving (g): 60
GL = 10

Food Name: Quinoa, cooked, refrigerated, reheated in
microwave for 1.5 min
GI = 53 ± 2
Serving (g): 150
GL = 13

Food Name: Raisin Bran Flax muffin, President's Choice® Blue
Menu™
GI = 52 ± 3
Serving (g): 70
GL = 17

Food Name: Raisins
GI = 49 ± 2
Serving (g): 28
GL = 10

Food Name: Raspberry 100% Pure Fruit spread, no added sugar
GI = 26 ± 2
Serving (g): 25
GL = 3

Food Name: Seeded bread
GI = 49 ± 2
Serving (g): 30
GL = 6

Food Name: Sliced Apples, canned, solid packed without juice
GI = 42 ± 2
Serving (g): 120
GL = 4

Food Name: Slim Fast™ French Vanilla ready-to-drink shake
GI = 37 ± 2
Serving (g): 250
GL = 10

Food Name: Smoothie drink soy, banana
GI = 30 ± 4
Serving (g): 250
GL = 7

Food Name: Smoothie drink, banana
GI = 30 ± 4
Serving (g): 250
GL = 8

Food Name: Smoothie drink, banana and strawberry, V8
Splash®
GI = 44 ± 4
Serving (g): 250
GL = 11

Food Name: Smoothie drink, mango
GI = 32 ± 4
Serving (g): 250
GL = 9

Food Name: Smoothie drink, raspberry
GI = 33 ± 4
Serving (g): 250
GL = 14

Food Name: Soy Crunch Multi-Grain Cereal, President's
Choice® Blue Menu™
GI = 47 ± 3
Serving (g): 30
GL = 9

Food Name: Soy milk, full-fat (3%), 120 mg calcium,
Calciforte
GI = 41 ± 3
Serving (g): 250
GL = 6

Food Name: Soy milk, full-fat (3%), Calciforte, 120 mg calcium,
with maltodextrin
GI = 36 ± 3
Serving (g): 250
GL = 6

Food Name: Soy milk, full-fat (3%), Original, 0 mg calcium, with maltodextrin
GI = 44 ± 3
Serving (g): 250
GL = 8

Food Name: Spaghetti bolognaise, home made
GI = 52 ± 2
Serving (g): 360
GL = 25

Food Name: Spaghetti, white, boiled
GI = 42 ± 3
Serving (g): 180
GL = 18

Food Name: Strawberries, fresh, raw
GI = 40 ± 3
Serving (g): 120
GL = 1

Food Name: Strawberry & wildberry dried fruit leather, Sunripe School Straps
GI = 40 ± 3
Serving (g): 30
GL = 8

Food Name: Strawberry & wildberry dried fruit leather, Sunripe School Straps
GI = 40 ± 3
Serving (g): 30
GL = 8

Food Name: Strawberry fruit leather

GI = 29 ± 3
Serving (g): 30
GL = 7

Food Name: SuperJuice Kickstart, containing apple juice, blueberry puree and banana puree
GI = 39 ± 3
Serving (g): 250
GL = 11

Food Name: Sushi, roasted sea algae, vinegar and rice
GI = 55 ± 3
Serving (g): 100
GL = 20

Food Name: Sushi, salmon
GI = 48 ± 3
Serving (g): 100
GL = 17

Food Name: Sweet and sour chicken with noodles, prepared convenience meal
GI = 41 ± 3
Serving (g): 300
GL = 21

Food Name: Sweet corn
GI = 55 ± 3
Serving (g): 80
GL = 9

Food Name: Sweet corn on the cob, boiled 20 min
GI = 48 ± 3
Serving (g): 80

GL = 8

Food Name: Sweet corn, cooked
GI = 52 ± 3
Serving (g): 150
GL = 17

Food Name: Sweet corn, frozen, reheated in microwave
GI = 47 ± 3
Serving (g): 150
GL = 16

Food Name: Sweet potato, boiled
GI = 44 ± 3
Serving (g): 150
GL = 11

Food Name: Tagliatelle, egg pasta, boiled in water for 7 min
GI = 46 ± 3
Serving (g): 180
GL = 20

Food Name: Tandoori chicken masala & rice convenience meal
GI = 45 ± 2
Serving (g): 300
GL = 27

Food Name: Tomato juice, no added sugar
GI = 33 ± 5
Serving (g): 250
GL = 3

Food Name: Tomato soup
GI = 38 ± 2

Serving (g): 250
GL = 6

Food Name: Tropical dried fruit snack
GI = 41 ± 4
Serving (g): 15
GL = 5

Food Name: Tuna fish bun
GI = 46 ± 4
Serving (g): 87
GL = 14

Food Name: V8 Splash®, tropical blend fruit drink
GI = 47 ± 3
Serving (g): 250
GL = 13

Food Name: V8® 100% vegetable juice
GI = 43 ± 3
Serving (g): 250
GL = 4

Food Name: Vanilla cake, made from packet mix with vanilla
frosting
GI = 42 ± 3
Serving (g): 111
GL = 24

Food Name: Vanilla pudding, instant, made from powder and
whole milk
GI = 40 ± 3
Serving (g): 100
GL = 6

Food Name: Vermicelli pasta, white, boiled
GI = 35 ± 3
Serving (g): 180
GL = 16

Food Name: White bread, homemade, frozen, defrosted and
toasted
GI = 52 ± 2
Serving (g): 30
GL = 7

Food Name: White rice, boiled
GI = 43 ± 4
Serving (g): 150
GL = 16

Food Name: White wheat flour bread, butter, cheese, regular
milk and fresh cucumber
GI = 55 ± 3
Serving (g): 200
GL = 37

Food Name: Whole-wheat bread with dried fruit
GI = 47 ± 3
Serving (g): 30
GL = 7

Food Name: Wholegrain water crackers with sesame seeds and
rosemary
GI = 53 ± 3
Serving (g): 25
GL = 8

Food Name: Wholemeal (whole wheat) bread

GI = 50 ± 3
Serving (g): 30
GL = 6

Food Name: Wild berry dried fruit snack
GI = 35 ± 2
Serving (g): 15
GL = 4

Food Name: Wild Oats Cluster Crunch Hazelnut Chocolate
breakfast cereal
GI = 43 ± 3
Serving (g): 30
GL = 8

Food Name: Xpress beverage, chocolate (soy bean, cereal and
legume extract drink with fructose)
GI = 39 ± 3
Serving (g): 250
GL = 13

Food Name: Yam
GI = 51 ± 3
Serving (g): 150
GL = 18

Chapter 3
MODERATE GLYCEMIC INDEX FOODS TABLES

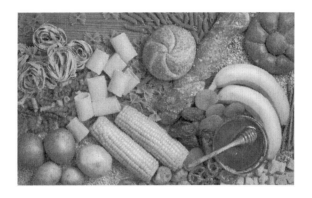

Moderate glycemic index category includes foods that have a
GI value in the range 56 to 69. This category includes corn,
white potatoes, white rice, sweet potatoes, breakfast cereals,
couscous.

Food Name: 100% Whole wheat Burger Buns
GI = 62 ± 2
Serving (g): 30
GL = 7

Food Name: 100% Whole wheat Hot Dog Rolls

GI = 62 ± 3
Serving (g): 30
GL = 7

Food Name: All-Bran Wheat Flakes™ breakfast cereal
GI = 60 ± 2
Serving (g): 30
GL = 12

Food Name: Apricot, coconut and honey muffin
GI = 60 ± 3
Serving (g): 50
GL = 16

Food Name: Apricot, raw
GI = 57 ± 2
Serving (g): 120
GL = 5

Food Name: Apricots, canned in light syrup
GI = 64 ± 3
Serving (g): 120
GL = 12

Food Name: Bagel, white bread
GI = 69 ± 3
Serving (g): 70
GL = 24

Food Name: Baked Beans in Tomato sauce, canned, reheated in
microwave for 1.5 min
GI = 57 ± 2
Serving (g): 150
GL = 13

Food Name: Banana, oat and honey muffin
GI = 65 ± 2
Serving (g): 50
GL = 17

Food Name: Banana, raw
GI = 58 ± 2
Serving (g): 120
GL = 13

Food Name: Barley flakes breakfast cereal
GI = 69 ± 4
Serving (g): 30
GL = 14

Food Name: Barley flour bread, 100% barley flour
GI = 67 ± 3
Serving (g): 30
GL = 9

Food Name: Barley, rolled
GI = 66 ± 3
Serving (g): 50
GL = 25

Food Name: Basmati, easy cook white rice, boiled 9 min
GI = 67 ± 3
Serving (g): 150
GL = 28

Food Name: Basmati, easy-cook white rice, consumed with 10 g margarine
GI = 68 ± 3
Serving (g): 150
GL = 28

Food Name: Basmati, white rice, organic, boiled 10 min
GI = 57 ± 3
Serving (g): 150
GL = 23

Food Name: Beer, Toohey's New
GI = 66 ± 3
Serving (g): 250
GL = 5

Food Name: Blueberry (Wild) 10-Grain muffin, President's
Choice® Blue Menu™
GI = 57 ± 3
Serving (g): 70
GL = 22

Food Name: Blueberry muffin
GI = 59 ± 3
Serving (g): 57
GL = 17

Food Name: Bran Flakes breakfast cereal
GI = 65 ± 3
Serving (g): 30
GL = 12

Food Name: Bran muffin
GI = 60 ± 3
Serving (g): 57
GL = 14

Food Name: Bread, flax, made from flax meal & wheat flour
GI = 67 ± 3
Serving (g): 30

GL = 8

Food Name: Breadfruit, raw
GI = 68 ± 2
Serving (g): 120
GL = 18

Food Name: Brown rice
GI = 66 ± 3
Serving (g): 150
GL = 22

Food Name: Buckwheat bread
GI = 67 ± 3
Serving (g): 30
GL = 13

Food Name: Carrot muffin
GI = 62 ± 3
Serving (g): 57
GL = 20

Food Name: Cereal biscuit (30 g), fruit flavor wheat biscuits
consumed with 125 mL skim milk
GI = 56 ± 2
Serving (g): 155
GL = 15

Food Name: Cherries, dark, raw, pitted
GI = 63 ± 3
Serving (g): 120
GL = 9

Food Name: Chicken and mushroom soup

GI = 69 ± 2
Serving (g): 250
GL = 13

Food Name: Chickpea flour bread, made from extruded
chickpea flour
GI = 67 ± 2
Serving (g): 30
GL = 8

Food Name: Classic French baguette bread with 10 g butter and
2 slices of ham (25 g)
GI = 59 ± 3
Serving (g): 100
GL = 25

Food Name: Clover honey, ratio of fructose: glucose, 1.09
GI = 69 ± 2
Serving (g): 25
GL = 15

Food Name: Coarse oat kernel bread, 80% intact oat kernels
and 20% white wheat flour
GI = 65 ± 3
Serving (g): 30
GL = 13

Food Name: Coca Cola®, soft drink
GI = 63 ± 3
Serving (g): 250
GL = 16

Food Name: Coco yam (Xanthosoma spp.), peeled, cubed,
boiled 30 min

GI = 61 ± 3
Serving (g): 150
GL = 28

Food Name: Cocoa Crunch cereal (30 g), consumed with 125 mL
skim milk
GI = 58 ± 3
Serving (g): 155
GL = 16

Food Name: Cordial, orange, reconstituted
GI = 66 ± 2
Serving (g): 250
GL = 13

Food Name: Corn pasta, gluten-free, Orgran brand
GI = 68 ± 3
Serving (g): 180
GL = 31

Food Name: Cornmeal + margarine
GI = 69 ± 3
Serving (g): 150
GL = 8

Food Name: Cornmeal porridge
GI = 68 ± 3
Serving (g): 150
GL = 9

Food Name: Cornmeal, boiled in salted water 2 min
GI = 68 ± 2
Serving (g): 150
GL = 9

Food Name: Cottage pie
GI = 65 ± 2
Serving (g): 300
GL = 22

Food Name: Couscous, boiled 5 min
GI = 63 ± 4
Serving (g): 150
GL = 21

Food Name: Cranberry juice cocktail
GI = 68 ± 3
Serving (g): 250
GL = 24

Food Name: Cranberry juice drink
GI = 56 ± 3
Serving (g): 250
GL = 16

Food Name: Creamed rice porridge
GI = 59 ± 3
Serving (g): 75
GL = 5

Food Name: Dates
GI = 62 ± 3
Serving (g): 60
GL = 21

Food Name: Digestives, cookies
GI = 59 ± 2
Serving (g): 25
GL = 9

Food Name: Fanta®, orange soft drink
GI = 68 ± 3
Serving (g): 250
GL = 23

Food Name: Fibre First Multi-Bran Cereal, President's Choice®
Blue Menu™
GI = 56 ± 3
Serving (g): 30
GL = 6

Food Name: Figs, dried, tenderised, Dessert Maid brand
GI = 61 ± 3
Serving (g): 60
GL = 16

Food Name: Fillet-O-Fish™ burger (fish patty, cheese and
tartare sauce on a burger bun)
GI = 66 ± 3
Serving (g): 128
GL = 20

Food Name: Flan cake (Weston's Bakery, Toronto, Canada)
GI = 65 ± 3
Serving (g): 70
GL = 31

Food Name: French baguette bread with butter and strawberry
jam
GI = 62 ± 3
Serving (g): 70
GL = 26

Food Name: Fruit and Fibre breakfast cereal

GI = 68 ± 3
Serving (g): 30
GL = 13

Food Name: Fruit loaf bread, sliced
GI = 57 ± 3
Serving (g): 30
GL = 9

Food Name: Fruit punch beverage
GI = 67 ± 3
Serving (g): 250
GL = 19

Food Name: Fruity-Bix™ bar, wheat biscuit cereal with dried
fruit and nuts with yoghurt coating
GI = 56 ± 3
Serving (g): 30
GL = 11

Food Name: Fusilli pasta twists, boiled 10 min in salted water
GI = 61 ± 3
Serving (g): 180
GL = 29

Food Name: Glucose, 50 g portion, consumed with 14.5 g
guar gum
GI = 62
Serving (g): 10
GL = 6

Food Name: Gnocchi, type not specified (Latina, Pillsbury
Australia Ltd, Mt. Waverley, Australia)
GI = 68 ± 4

Serving (g): 180

GL = 33

Food Name: Granola Clusters breakfast cereal, Original, low fat, President's Choice® Blue Menu™

GI = 63 ± 2

Serving (g): 30

GL = 14

Food Name: Grany Rush Apricot, digestive cookies

GI = 62 ± 2

Serving (g): 30

GL = 12

Food Name: Grapes, black, Waltham Cross

GI = 59 ± 2

Serving (g): 120

GL = 11

Food Name: Hamburger (beef patty, ketchup, pickle, onion and mustard on a burger bun)

GI = 66 ± 4

Serving (g): 95

GL = 17

Food Name: Hamburger bun

GI = 61 ± 3

Serving (g): 30

GL = 9

Food Name: Happiness™ bread, cinnamon, raisin, pecan bread

GI = 63 ± 2

Serving (g): 30

GL = 9

Food Name: Healthwise™ for bowel health breakfast cereal
GI = 66 ± 2
Serving (g): 30
GL = 12

Food Name: Honey, Commercial Blend (38% fructose)
GI = 62 ± 2
Serving (g): 25
GL = 11

Food Name: Honey, Pure
GI = 58 ± 3
Serving (g): 25
GL = 12

Food Name: Honey, Pure
GI = 58 ± 3
Serving (g): 25
GL = 12

Food Name: Honey, Salvation Jane (32% fructose)
GI = 64 ± 3
Serving (g): 25
GL = 10

Food Name: Hunger Filler™, whole grain bread
GI = 59 ± 2
Serving (g): 30
GL = 7

Food Name: Ice cream (half vanilla, half chocolate),
regular/type not specified
GI = 57 ± 2
Serving (g): 50

GL = 6

Food Name: Instant porridge
GI = 69 ± 2
Serving (g): 250
GL = 14

Food Name: Kiwi fruit
GI = 58 ± 2
Serving (g): 120
GL = 7

Food Name: Lean beef burger (lean beef patty, tomato, mixed
lettuce, cheese, onion and sauce on a burger bun)
GI = 66 ± 4
Serving (g): 164
GL = 17

Food Name: Lentil and cauliflower cury with rice
GI = 60 ± 2
Serving (g): 300
GL = 25

Food Name: Low-fat yoghurt, peach melba
GI = 56 ± 2
Serving (g): 200
GL = 16

Food Name: Low-fat yoghurt, strawberry
GI = 61 ± 2
Serving (g): 200
GL = 18

Food Name: LU Petit Dejeuner Chocolate & Cereals cookies

GI = 58 ± 3
Serving (g): 50
GL = 20

Food Name: Macaroni, boiled
GI = 56 ± 2
Serving (g): 180
GL = 27

Food Name: Mars Bar® (M&M/Mars, USA)
GI = 68 ± 3
Serving (g): 60
GL = 27

Food Name: Marshmallows
GI = 62 ± 2
Serving (g): 30
GL = 15

Food Name: McChicken™ burger (chicken patty, lettuce,
mayonnaise on a burger bun)
GI = 66 ± 2
Serving (g): 186
GL = 26

Food Name: Oro cookies
GI = 61 ± 3
Serving (g): 40
GL = 21

Food Name: Pastry
GI = 59 ± 3
Serving (g): 57
GL = 15

Food Name: Peach, canned in heavy syrup
GI = 64 ± 3
Serving (g): 120
GL = 12

Food Name: Peach, raw
GI = 56 ± 2
Serving (g): 120
GL = 5

Food Name: Pineapple, raw
GI = 66 ± 2
Serving (g): 120
GL = 6

Food Name: Pita bread, white
GI = 67 ± 2
Serving (g): 30
GL = 10

Food Name: Pita bread, white (Sainsbury's, UK), with 5 g
margarine
GI = 67 ± 2
Serving (g): 30
GL = 10

Food Name: Pita bread, wholemeal
GI = 56 ± 2
Serving (g): 30
GL = 8

Food Name: Pizza, cheese
GI = 60 ± 2
Serving (g): 100

GL = 16

Food Name: Porridge, made from rolled oats
GI = 63 ± 2
Serving (g): 250
GL = 19

Food Name: Potato, type not specified, boiled
GI = 66 ± 2
Serving (g): 150
GL = 13

Food Name: Potato, white with skin, baked, consumed with 10 g margarine
GI = 69 ± 2
Serving (g): 150
GL = 19

Food Name: Potato, white, cooked
GI = 61 ± 2
Serving (g): 150
GL = 16

Food Name: Probiotic yoghurt drink, cranberry
GI = 56 ± 2
Serving (g): 250
GL = 17
Food Name: Raisins
GI = 66 ± 2
Serving (g): 60
GL = 28

Food Name: Soy Tasty™ breakfast cereal (flaked grains, soy nuts, dried fruit)

GI = 60 ± 2
Serving (g): 30
GL = 12

Food Name: Spaghetti, white, durum wheat, boiled 20 min
GI = 58 ± 3
Serving (g): 180
GL = 26

Food Name: Special K™ breakfast cereal
GI = 69 ± 3
Serving (g): 30
GL = 14

Food Name: Sugar (Sucrose), 100 g portion
GI = 65
Serving (g): 10
GL = 7

Food Name: Sunflower and barley bread
GI = 57 ± 2
Serving (g): 30
GL = 6

Food Name: Sweet corn
GI = 62 ± 2
Serving (g): 80
GL = 11

Food Name: Sweet corn, boiled
GI = 60 ± 2
Serving (g): 80
GL = 11

Food Name: Traditional French baguette (prepared with wheat
flour, water, salt and 20 g yeast)
GI = 69 ± 2
Serving (g): 30
GL = 12

Food Name: Vegetable soup
GI = 60 ± 2
Serving (g): 250
GL = 11

Food Name: White bread with added wheatgerm and fiber
GI = 59 ± 2
Serving (g): 30
GL = 6

Food Name: White bread with butter
GI = 59 ± 2
Serving (g): 100
GL = 28

Food Name: White bread, fresh, toasted
GI = 63 ± 2
Serving (g): 30
GL = 8

Food Name: White bread, homemade, fresh, toasted
GI = 66 ± 2
Serving (g): 30
GL = 9

Food Name: White bread, wheat flour
GI = 69 ± 2
Serving (g): 30

GL = 10

Food Name: White bread, wheat flour, frozen, defrosted and toasted
GI = 64 ± 2
Serving (g): 30
GL = 8

Food Name: Wholemeal bread, stoneground flour
GI = 59 ± 1
Serving (g): 30
GL = 7

Food Name: Yoghurt, black cherry
GI = 67 ± 3
Serving (g): 200
GL = 8

Food Name: Yoghurt, bourbon vanilla
GI = 64 ± 3
Serving (g): 200
GL = 20

Food Name: Yoghurt, lemon curd
GI = 67 ± 3
Serving (g): 200
GL = 30

Food Name: Yoghurt, peach melba
GI = 57 ± 3
Serving (g): 200
GL = 18

Chapter 4
HIGH GLYCEMIC INDEX
FOODS TABLES

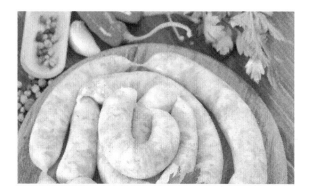

High glycemic index category contains foods that have a GI
value of 70 or higher. This category includes foods that are bad
to health and cause high spikes in blood sugar level. Foods that
fall in this category should be avoided like packaged breakfast
cereals, white bread, doughnuts, bagels, most crackers, rice
cakes, croissants.

Food Name : 15 g Oat bran (containing 2 g ß-glucan), consumed
as a drink mixed with 41g glucose and water
GI = 84 ± 3
Serving(g): 10

GL = 2

Food Name : Bagel, white, frozen (Lender's Bakery, Montreal, Canada)
GI = 72 ± 3
Serving(g): 70
GL = 25

Food Name : Baguette, white, plain
GI = 95 ± 2
Serving(g): 30
GL = 14

Food Name : Barley flour bread, made from 50% wheat flour and 50% coarse sieved barley flour
GI = 74 ± 3
Serving(g): 30
GL = 12

Food Name : Barquette Abricot cookies
GI = 71 ± 4
Serving(g): 40
GL = 23

Food Name : Blackbread, Riga
GI = 76 ± 3
Serving(g): 30
GL = 10

Food Name : Bran Flakes™ breakfast cereal
GI = 74 ± 4
Serving(g): 30
GL = 13

Food Name : Bread stuffing, Paxo
GI = 74 ± 3
Serving(g): 30
GL = 16

Food Name : Breadfruit roasted on preheated charcoal
GI = 72 ± 3
Serving(g): 120
GL = 20

Food Name : Broken rice, white, cooked in rice cooker
GI = 86 ± 3
Serving(g): 150
GL = 37

Food Name : Brown rice
GI = 87 ± 2
Serving(g): 150
GL = 29

Food Name : Brown rice, boiled in excess water for 25 min,
SunRice brand
GI = 72 ± 3
Serving(g): 150
GL = 29

Food Name : Brown rice, boiled in excess water for 25 min,
SunRice brand
GI = 72 ± 3
Serving(g): 150
GL = 29

Food Name : Cheerios™ breakfast cereal
GI = 74 ± 4

Serving(g): 30
GL = 15

Food Name : Chicken Tandoori Deli Choice white French roll
white bread
GI = 78 ± 3
Serving(g): 270
GL = 44

Food Name : Chocapic™ breakfast cereal, wheat-based flaked
cereal
GI = 70 ± 4
Serving(g): 30
GL = 17

Food Name : Coco Pops™ breakfast cereal (cocoa flavored
puffed rice)
GI = 77 ± 4
Serving(g): 30
GL = 20

Food Name : Corn Bran™ breakfast cereal
GI = 75 ± 4
Serving(g): 30
GL = 15

Food Name : Corn Chex™ breakfast cereal
GI = 83 ± 4
Serving(g): 30
GL = 21

Food Name : Corn pasta, gluten-free, Orgran brand
GI = 78 ± 2
Serving(g): 180

GL = 32

Food Name : Corn Pops™ breakfast cereal
GI = 80 ± 4
Serving(g): 30
GL = 21

Food Name : Cornflakes breakfast cereal
GI = 79 ± 4
Serving(g): 30
GL = 20

Food Name : Cornflakes breakfast cereal (Kellogg's, France)
GI = 93 ± 4
Serving(g): 30
GL = 25

Food Name : Cornflakes breakfast cereal consumed with 150
mL semi-skimmed milk
GI = 93 ± 4
Serving(g): 30
GL = 23

Food Name : Cornflakes, Crunchy Nut™ breakfast cereal
GI = 72 ± 4
Serving(g): 30
GL = 17

Food Name : Cornflakes™ breakfast cereal
GI = 77 ± 4
Serving(g): 30
GL = 19

Food Name : Cornflakes™ breakfast cereal

GI = 80 ± 4
Serving(g): 30
GL = 21

Food Name : Cornflakes™ breakfast cereal (Kellogg's Inc.,
Canada)
GI = 86 ± 4
Serving(g): 30
GL = 22

Food Name : Cornflakes™ breakfast cereal (Kellogg's, USA)
GI = 92 ± 4
Serving(g): 30
GL = 24

Food Name : Cotton honey, ratio of fructose:glucose, 1.03
GI = 74 ± 2
Serving(g): 25
GL = 16

Food Name : Crunchy Nut Cornflakes™ bar
GI = 72 ± 4
Serving(g): 30
GL = 19

Food Name : Crunchy Nut Cornflakes™ bar
GI = 72 ± 3
Serving(g): 30
GL = 19

Food Name : Cupcake, strawberry-iced, Squiggles
GI = 73 ± 3
Serving(g): 38
GL = 19

Food Name : Doughnut, wheat dough, deep-fried
GI = 75 ± 2
Serving(g): 50
GL = 15

Food Name : Fiber White™ bread
GI = 77 ± 2
Serving(g): 30
GL = 11

Food Name : French baguette bread with chocolate spread
GI = 72 ± 3
Serving(g): 70
GL = 27

Food Name : French bread, fermented with yeast
GI = 81 ± 2
Serving(g): 30
GL = 13

Food Name : Fruit and cinnamon bread
GI = 71 ± 3
Serving(g): 30
GL = 11

Food Name : Fruit and cinnamon bread
GI = 71 ± 2
Serving(g): 30
GL = 11

Food Name : Gluten Free Multigrain bread
GI = 79 ± 3
Serving(g): 30
GL = 10

Food Name : Gluten-free buckwheat bread, made with
buckwheat meal & rice flour
GI = 72 ± 2
Serving(g): 30
GL = 8

Food Name : Gluten-free white bread, unsliced (gluten-free
wheat starch)
GI = 71 ± 3
Serving(g): 30
GL = 10

Food Name : Golden Wheats™ breakfast cereal
GI = 71 ± 2
Serving(g): 30
GL = 16

Food Name : Granola Clusters breakfast cereal, Raisin &
Almond, low fat, President's Choice® Blue Menu™
GI = 70 ± 4
Serving(g): 30
GL = 15

Food Name : Grapenuts™ breakfast cereal
GI = 75 ± 4
Serving(g): 30
GL = 16

Food Name : Honey Goldies™ wheat biscuits with additional
ingredients
GI = 72 ± 4
Serving(g): 30
GL = 15

Food Name : Honey Rice Bubbles™ breakfast cereal
GI = 77 ± 3
Serving(g): 30
GL = 20

Food Name : Honey Smacks™ breakfast cereal
GI = 71 ± 4
Serving(g): 30
GL = 16

Food Name : Honey, Commercial Blend (28% fructose), NSW
blend
GI = 72 ± 3
Serving(g): 25
GL = 9

Food Name : Instant oat cereal porridge prepared with water
GI = 83 ± 3
Serving(g): 250
GL = 30

Food Name : Instant oat porridge, cooked in microwave with
water
GI = 82 ± 3
Serving(g): 250
GL = 20

Food Name : Japanese Wasabi & Honey Rice & Corn Crisps,
GI = 82 ± 3
Serving(g): 50
GL = 32

Food Name : Jelly beans, assorted colors (Allen's, Nestlé, Australia)
GI = 80 ± 4

Serving(g): 30
GL = 22

Food Name : Jelly beans, assorted colors (Savings, Grocery Holdings, Tooronga, Australia)
GI = 76 ± 3
Serving(g): 30
GL = 21

Food Name : Morning Coffee™ cookies
GI = 79 ± 4
Serving(g): 25
GL = 15

Food Name : Muesli
GI = 86 ± 4
Serving(g): 30
GL = 18

Food Name : Multigrain bread, with 5 g maragrine
GI = 80 ± 3
Serving(g): 30
GL = 8

Food Name : Pancakes, prepared from wheat flour
GI = 80 ± 3
Serving(g): 80
GL = 16

Food Name : Pikelets, Golden brand
GI = 85 ± 3
Serving(g): 40
GL = 18

Food Name : Pizza, plain baked dough, served with parmesan
cheese and tomato sauce
GI = 80 ± 2
Serving(g): 100
GL = 22

Food Name : Potato, type not specified, boiled in salted water
GI = 76 ± 2
Serving(g): 150
GL = 26

Food Name : Potato, type not specified, peeled, boiled
GI = 85 ± 2
Serving(g): 150
GL = 26

Food Name : Pumpkin Soup, creamy, Heinz® Very Special™,
with pumpkin, cream, potatoes
GI = 76 ± 2
Serving(g): 250
GL = 14

Food Name : Pumpkin, boiled in salted water
GI = 75 ± 2
Serving(g): 80
GL = 3

Food Name : Raspberry Fruit bar, fat-free, President's Choice®
Blue Menu™ (Loblaw Brands Limited, Canada)
GI = 74 ± 2
Serving(g): 40
GL = 23

Food Name : Real Fruit Bars, strawberry (Uncle Toby's, Australia)
GI = 90 ± 3
Serving(g): 30
GL = 23

Food Name : Rice milk drink, low-fat, Australia's Own Natural™
GI = 92 ± 3
Serving(g): 250
GL = 29

Food Name : Rice Pops™, with 125 mL semi-skimmed milk
GI = 80 ± 4
Serving(g): 30
GL = 20

Food Name : Rice porridge
GI = 88 ± 3
Serving(g): 150
GL = 13

Food Name : Rockmelon/Cantaloupe, raw
GI = 70 ± 2
Serving(g): 120
GL = 4

Food Name : Special K™ breakfast cereal, made from rice
GI = 84 ± 4
Serving(g): 30
GL = 20

Food Name : Strawberry processed fruit bars, Real Fruit Bars
GI = 90 ± 2

Serving(g): 30

GL = 23

Food Name : Watermelon, raw

GI = 80 ± 2

Serving(g): 120

GL = 5

Food Name : Wheat based cereal biscuit, wheat biscuits (plain flaked wheat)

GI = 72 ± 4

Serving(g): 30

GL = 14

Food Name : Wheat-bites™ breakfast cereal

GI = 72 ± 3

Serving(g): 30

GL = 18

Food Name : White bread, wheat flour

GI = 78 ± 3

Serving(g): 30

GL = 12

Food Name : Wholemeal (whole wheat) bread

GI = 71 ± 2

Serving(g): 30

GL = 9

HEALTH AND NUTRITION RESOURCES

American Academy of Family Physicians (www.familydoctor.org)

American Academy of Pediatrics (www.aacap.org)

American Diabetes Association (www.diabetes.org)

American Heart Association (www.americanheart.org)

Easy Keto Diet (www.easyketodiet.net)

Glycemic Index database (https://www.easyketodiet.net/glycemic-index-counter/)

Centers for Disease Control and Prevention (www.cdc.gov/healthyweight)

Cooking Light (www.cookinglight.com)

Eating Well (www.eatingwell.com)

eMedicine Health (www.emedicinehealth.com)

Fruits and Vegetables Matter (www.fruitsandveggiesmatter.gov)

Health (www.health.com)

Hormone Foundation (www.hormone.org)

Jillian Michaels (www.jillianmichaels.com)

Joy Bauer (www.joybauer.com)

Mayo Clinic (www.mayoclinic.com)

Medline Plus (www.nlm.nih.gov/medlineplus)

My Fitness Pal (www.myfitnesspal.com)
National Cancer Institute (www.cancer.gov)
National Digestive Diseases Information Clearinghouse
(www.digestive.niddk.nih.gov)
National Heart, Lung, Blood Institute (www.nhlbi.nih.gov)
National Institute on Aging (www.nia.nih.gov)
National Institutes of Health (http://health.nih.gov)
Nutrition.gov (www.nutrition.gov)
Prevention (www.prevention.com)

Printed in Great Britain
by Amazon